Nurturing Your Mind

A Comprehensive Guide to Women's Mental Health and Self-Care

Rita J. Alexander

Contents

Introduction

Welcome to Nurturing Your Mind: A Comprehensive Guide to Women's Mental Health and Self-Care. Whether you are a woman struggling with mental health challenges, looking to enhance your overall well-being, or simply seeking to maintain a healthy mind and body, this book is for you.

As women, we face unique challenges and stressors in our daily lives that can take a toll on our mental health. From societal pressures to family responsibilities to personal expectations, it can feel like we're constantly juggling multiple roles and struggling to keep up. But despite the challenges, it's essential to prioritize our mental health and well-being.

Nurturing Your Mind is more than just a self-help book. It's a roadmap to empowering yourself and reclaiming control over your life. In this book, you'll find evidence-based strategies and practical advice to help you build resilience, manage stress, and overcome common mental health challenges.

We'll start by exploring the connection between the mind and body and how simple self-care practices can profoundly impact your mental health. We'll also delve into the importance of building a support system, seeking professional help when necessary, and overcoming common mental health challenges.

By the end of this book, you'll better understand women's

mental health and feel empowered to take action and prioritize your well-being. Remember, you are not alone in your struggles; there is always help and hope available.

So, let's get started on this journey of self-discovery, healing, and growth together.

Why Mental Health and Self-Care Are So Important for Women

Mental health and self-care are crucial for women because they play a fundamental role in overall well-being, quality of life, and ability to function effectively. Cognitive health refers to our emotional, psychological, and social well-being. It includes coping with stress, maintaining healthy relationships, and making decisions that align with our values and goals. Self-care, conversely, encompasses all the activities and practices we engage in to maintain and improve our physical, mental, and emotional health.

Unfortunately, women are often disproportionately affected by mental health issues. Study shows that females are more likely than males to experience anxiety, depression, post-traumatic stress disorder (PTSD), eating disorders, and other mental health conditions. Additionally, women may face unique stressors and challenges, such as gender-based violence, discrimination, and societal expectations related to gender roles, which can further impact mental health.

This is why mental health and self-care are so important for women. By prioritizing mental health and engaging in self-care practices, women can improve their overall well-being and quality of life and build resilience and coping skills to manage stress and challenges. This can positive ripple effect on other areas of life, including relationships, work, and personal growth.

Engaging in self-care practices can also help women develop self-awareness and self-compassion, essential mental health components. By caring for ourselves and meeting our needs, we can cultivate a more profound understanding of self-respect, self-esteem, and self-love.

Ultimately, mental health and self-care are critical for women because they enable us to live life fully and reach our full potential. By prioritizing our mental health and well-being, we can be our best selves and make meaningful contributions to the world.

Chapter 1: Understanding Women's Mental Health

Understanding women's mental health is crucial for promoting overall well-being and ensuring women have access to the support and resources they need to manage their mental health effectively. Women's mental health refers to their emotional, psychological, and social well-being, including their ability to cope with stress, maintain healthy relationships, and make decisions that align with their values and goals.

Women may experience a range of mental health challenges, including depression, anxiety, bipolar disorder, post-traumatic stress disorder (PTSD), eating disorders, and substance abuse. Additionally, women may be more susceptible to certain mental health conditions, such as postpartum depression and premenstrual dysphoric disorder (PMDD), directly related to reproductive health.

Several factors can influence women's mental health, including biology, environment, and social and cultural influences. For example, hormonal changes during puberty, pregnancy, and menopause can affect women's mental health, as can environmental factors like stress, trauma, and socioeconomic status. Social and cultural factors can also impact women's mental health, such as discrimination, gender roles, and societal expectations.

It's important to note that women's mental health is not a one-size-fits-all issue. Women from different backgrounds and experiences may have unique mental health needs and challenges. Understanding these differences and a holistic approach to mental health is critical to promoting well-being and providing practical support.

Some strategies that can help promote women's mental health include engaging in self-care practices, seeking professional support when necessary, building a solid support network, and advocating for mental health policies and resources. Additionally, reducing stigma around mental health and encouraging open communication can help create a more supportive and accepting environment for women with mental health challenges.

In summary, understanding women's mental health is crucial for promoting overall well-being and ensuring women have access to the support and resources they need to manage their mental health effectively. By recognizing women's unique challenges and needs, we can work towards a more equitable and supportive world for all.

Common Mental Health Challenges Faced by Women

Women face various mental health challenges that can impact their overall well-being, relationships, and ability to function effectively. Some of the most common mental health challenges faced by women include:

1. Anxiety disorders: Females are twice as likely as males to experience anxiety disorders, including generalized anxiety disorder, panic disorder, and obsessive-compulsive disorder. These conditions can cause excessive worry, fear, and avoidance behaviors that interfere with daily life.

2. Depression: Depression is a common mental health challenge for women, with an estimated one in four women experiencing depression at some point. Depression can cause feelings of sadness, hopelessness, and worthlessness, as well as physical symptoms like fatigue and changes in appetite and sleep patterns.

3. Eating disorders: Eating disturbances, such as anorexia nervosa, bulimia nervosa, and binge eating disorder, are more common in women than men. These conditions can cause distorted thinking about food, body image, and physical health complications.

4. Post-traumatic stress disorder (PTSD): Women are more

likely than men to experience PTSD, which can result from experiencing or witnessing a traumatic event. Symptoms can include flashbacks, avoidance behaviors, and hypervigilance.

5. Substance abuse: Women may be more susceptible to substance abuse and addiction than men and may also face unique challenges related to stigma and barriers to treatment.

6. Reproductive health-related mental health challenges: Women may experience mental health challenges related to reproductive health, such as premenstrual dysphoric disorder (PMDD), postpartum depression, and perimenopausal depression.

It's important to note that women's mental health challenges are not limited to these conditions and that they may also experience unique mental health challenges related to their experiences and backgrounds. Seeking professional support, engaging in self-care practices, building a strong support network, and advocating for mental health policies and resources can help address these challenges and promote overall well-being.

Stigma and Barriers to Treatment

Stigma and barriers to treatment are major obstacles that can prevent women from accessing the mental health care they need. Stigma refers to negative attitudes and beliefs leading to discrimination and social exclusion. In contrast, barriers to treatment refer to practical challenges that can make it difficult for women to access mental health care.

Stigma can take many forms, including societal stereotypes and prejudices and self-stigma, which occurs when individuals internalize negative beliefs about mental illness and feel ashamed or embarrassed to seek help. Stigma can prevent women from seeking treatment for mental health challenges, as they may fear judgment or discrimination from others. This can be particularly problematic in communities where mental illness is stigmatized or seeking help for mental health challenges is viewed as a sign of weakness.

Barriers to treatment can also prevent women from accessing mental health care. These barriers can include a lack of access to affordable or convenient mental health services, issues related to insurance coverage, and the availability of trained mental health professionals. Women may also face practical barriers related to caregiving responsibilities or transportation, making attending appointments or engaging in treatment difficult.

Addressing stigma and barriers to treatment is crucial for

promoting women's mental health and ensuring they have access to the care and resources they need. Addressing stigma can include increasing public education and awareness about mental health, promoting open communication, and reducing stereotypes and prejudices. Barriers to treatment can be addressed by increasing access to affordable and convenient mental health services, expanding insurance coverage for mental health care, and increasing the availability of trained mental health professionals in underserved areas.

By addressing stigma and barriers to treatment, we can help ensure that women can access the care and resources they need to manage their mental health effectively, promoting overall well-being and quality of life.

The Importance of Early Intervention

Early intervention is critical in promoting women's mental health and preventing the development of more severe mental health challenges. This is because mental health challenges often develop gradually and can become more difficult to treat if left unaddressed.

Early intervention can involve a range of strategies, including:

1. Screening: Regular screening for mental health challenges can help identify potential issues early on and ensure that women receive the care and resources they need to manage their mental health effectively.

2. Education and awareness: Educating women about the signs and symptoms of mental health challenges and the importance of seeking early help can ensure that women are more likely to recognize potential issues and seek help when needed.

3. Prevention programs: Prevention programs, such as those focused on reducing stress, building resilience, and promoting healthy coping strategies, can help prevent mental health challenges from developing in the first place.

4. Treatment: Providing prompt treatment and support to women experiencing mental health challenges can help prevent those challenges from becoming more severe and difficult to treat. This can include a range of

interventions, such as therapy, medication, and support groups.

Early intervention is particularly important for women at higher risk for mental health challenges, such as those who have experienced trauma, those with a relative history of mental illness, or those going through major life transitions like pregnancy or menopause.

We can assist in ensuring women have the tools and support they need to maintain their well-being, develop resilience, and succeed in all aspects of their life by emphasizing early intervention and proactive efforts to promote women's mental health.

Chapter 2: The Mind-Body Connection

The mind-body connection is the relationship between our thoughts, emotions, and physical health. It is a fundamental concept in the mental health field and is based on the idea that our thoughts and emotions can profoundly impact our physical well-being.

Research has shown that the mind-body connection is complex and multifaceted, with various factors influencing the relationship between our thoughts, emotions, and physical health. For example, stress and anxiety can lead to physical symptoms like headaches, fatigue, and digestive issues. At the same time, positive emotions like joy and gratitude can improve our overall sense of well-being and boost our immune system.

The mind-body connection is also important when managing mental health challenges. For example, engaging in physical activity can be a powerful way to boost mood, reduce stress, and improve overall well-being. Similarly, practicing mindfulness meditation can help reduce symptoms of anxiety and depression while promoting feelings of calm and relaxation.

Overall, the mind-body connection highlights the importance of a holistic approach to mental health and well-being. By recognizing the interplay between our thoughts, emotions, and physical health, we can take proactive steps to support our overall health and well-being, reducing the risk of mental health challenges and promoting a greater sense of balance and harmony.

How Your Mind Affects Your Body and Vice Versa

The mind and body are not separate entities but are instead deeply interconnected. Our thoughts, emotions, and behaviors can profoundly impact our physical health, while our physical health can also impact our mental well-being.

For example, when we experience stress, our body releases hormones like cortisol and adrenaline. These hormones can increase heart, blood, and respiratory rates, preparing us for the fight-or-flight response. However, if we experience chronic stress, this constant activation of the stress response can negatively affect our physical health, including an increased risk for cardiovascular disease, diabetes, and other chronic health conditions.

Conversely, physical health can also impact our mental well-being. For example, regular physical activity has been shown to improve mood, reduce symptoms of anxiety and depression, and boost overall well-being. Similarly, eating a healthy diet and getting enough sleep can also positively impact our mental health.

The mind-body connection also highlights the importance of taking a holistic approach to health and wellness. By recognizing the interplay between our thoughts, emotions, and physical health, we can take proactive steps to support our overall well-being, reducing the risk of mental health challenges and promoting a greater sense of balance and harmony in our lives.

This can involve a range of strategies, including practicing mindfulness meditation, engaging in regular physical activity, and seeking treatment and support for mental health challenges when needed.

The Benefits of Mind-Body Practices for Mental Health and Self-Care

Mind-body practices focus on the relationship between the mind and body to promote health and well-being. These practices have been used for centuries in various cultures and traditions and have gained increasing recognition in recent years for their mental health benefits.

One of the primary benefits of mind-body practices is their ability to reduce stress and promote relaxation. Techniques like yoga, tai chi, and meditation have been shown to reduce cortisol levels and improve overall mood, reducing symptoms of anxiety and depression. Additionally, these practices can help increase self-awareness and self-compassion, promoting a greater sense of emotional balance and resilience.

Mind-body practices can also be effective for managing chronic pain. Techniques like mindfulness meditation and guided imagery can help reduce pain perception, allowing individuals to manage their symptoms more effectively and improve their overall quality of life.

Another benefit of mind-body practices is their ability to improve sleep quality. Meditation or gentle yoga before bedtime can help calm the mind and promote relaxation, reducing sleep disturbances and improving overall sleep quality.

Mind-body practices can be a powerful tool for promoting mental health and self-care. By helping individuals manage stress, reduce symptoms of anxiety and depression, and improve overall well-being, these practices can support individuals in achieving greater balance and harmony in their lives.

Chapter 3: Self-Care Strategies for Women

Self-care is a critical component of overall health and well-being. It involves taking proactive steps to care for oneself physically, mentally, and emotionally. For women, who often juggle multiple responsibilities and demands, self-care is especially important to maintain health and prevent burnout.

There are many self-care strategies that women can incorporate into their daily lives. Physical self-care includes regular exercise, sleeping well, and eating a healthy diet. Recurring physical activity can help reduce stress and boost mood, while getting enough sleep and eating a balanced diet can help support overall physical health and well-being.

Mental and emotional self-care strategies include meditation, journaling, and time in nature. Meditation and mindfulness practices can help reduce symptoms of anxiety and depression, while journaling can help increase self-awareness and promote emotional processing. Spending time in nature has also been shown to positively impact mental health and well-being, promoting feelings of calm and reducing stress.

Other self-care strategies include engaging in hobbies and activities that bring joy and relaxation, connecting with supportive friends and family, and setting healthy boundaries to manage stress and prevent burnout. These strategies can help promote overall well-being and resilience, reducing the risk of mental health challenges and promoting greater balance and harmony in one's life.

Incorporating self-care strategies into daily life can be challenging, especially for women with competing demands and responsibilities. However, taking even small steps towards self-care can significantly impact overall health and well-being, reducing stress and promoting a greater sense of balance and harmony in one's life.

Self-Care Essentials: Sleep, Nutrition, Exercise, and Hydration

Self-care essentials are the basic components of caring for oneself physically and mentally. They include sleep, nutrition, exercise, and hydration, all essential for maintaining good health and well-being.

Sleep is one of the most important self-care essentials. Getting enough quality sleep is essential for maintaining physical and mental health. Sleep helps the body repair and regenerate, and it's also critical for cognitive functioning, emotional regulation, and overall mood. For adults, it is recommended to get 7-9 hours of sleep per night.

Nutrition is another important self-care essential. Eating a healthy and balanced diet rich in whole foods, fruits, vegetables, and lean protein is critical for maintaining physical and mental health. A nourishing diet can help reduce the risk of chronic diseases like diabetes, heart disease, and certain types of cancer while supporting overall cognitive functioning and mood.

Exercise is also an essential component of self-care. Regular physical activity can help improve cardiovascular health, reduce the risk of chronic diseases, and promote overall physical and mental well-being. Exercise has also been shown to positively impact mood, reducing symptoms of depression and anxiety.

Hydration is the final self-care essential. Drinking enough water is essential for maintaining proper bodily functions and overall health. Water helps control body temperature, transport nutrients, and remove waste from the body. Staying hydrated can also help improve cognitive functioning and mood.

Overall, prioritizing self-care essentials like sleep, nutrition, exercise, and hydration can significantly impact overall health and well-being. Incorporating these practices into daily life can help reduce the risk of chronic diseases, promote physical and mental well-being, and support a greater sense of balance and harmony.

Other Self-Care Practices: Journaling, Mindfulness, Gratitude, and More

In addition to the self-care essentials of sleep, nutrition, exercise, and hydration, many other self-care practices can help support mental health and well-being. These practices can help reduce stress, promote a sense of calm and balance, and increase overall feelings of well-being.

Journaling is one self-care practice that can help increase self-awareness, promote emotional processing, and reduce stress. By writing down thoughts, feelings, and experiences, individuals can gain insight into their own thought patterns and behaviors and healthily process difficult emotions.

Mindfulness is another self-care practice that involves being present in the moment and cultivating non-judgmental awareness of one's thoughts and emotions. Mindfulness techniques, such as meditation, can help reduce symptoms of anxiety and depression, increase feelings of calm and relaxation, and improve overall mood and well-being.

Gratitude is also an important self-care practice. Cultivating gratitude and appreciation for the good things in life can help shift focus away from negative thoughts and emotions, reduce stress, and increase overall well-being. Practicing gratitude can involve keeping a gratitude journal, making a daily gratitude list, or simply appreciating the good things in life.

Other self-care practices may include engaging in creative hobbies or activities like art or music, spending time in nature, setting healthy boundaries, connecting with supportive friends and family, or practicing self-compassion and self-forgiveness. These practices can all help support mental health and well-being, reducing stress, promoting a greater sense of balance and harmony, and increasing overall well-being.

Overall, incorporating self-care practices like journaling, mindfulness, gratitude, and others into daily life can significantly impact mental health and well-being. By taking time to care for oneself physically, mentally, and emotionally, individuals can promote greater balance and harmony, reduce the risk of mental health challenges, and increase overall well-being.

Creating a Self-Care Plan That Works for You

Creating a self-care plan that works for you is important in promoting mental health and well-being. A self-care plan can help you identify the activities and practices that are most helpful for you and incorporate them into your daily routine in a way that feels manageable and sustainable.

To create a self-care plan, identify your specific needs and priorities. Consider what activities or practices make you feel most calm, centered, and grounded, as well as what challenges or stressors you may face. This could involve taking a self-assessment or inventory of your physical, emotional, and mental well-being and identifying areas where you may need additional support or attention.

Next, brainstorm a list of self-care activities and practices that align with your needs and priorities. This could include exercise, meditation, spending time in nature, connecting with loved ones, or engaging in creative hobbies or activities.

Once you have identified potential self-care activities, consider how you can incorporate them into your daily routine in a manageable and sustainable way. This could involve scheduling time for self-care activities on your calendar, setting realistic goals and expectations, and prioritizing self-care as an important aspect of your overall well-being.

It is also helpful to track your progress and reflect on the most helpful activities or practices. This could involve keeping a self-care journal, tracking your mood and energy levels, or seeking feedback and support from others.

Remember that self-care is a highly individualized process, and what works for one person may not work for another. It is important to be patient and compassionate with yourself as you explore different self-care practices and find what works best for you. By creating a self-care plan tailored to your unique needs and priorities, you can promote greater balance and harmony in your life, reduce the risk of mental health challenges, and increase overall well-being.

Chapter 4: Building a Support System

Building a support system is important to maintaining good mental health and promoting self-care. A support system is a network of people who provide emotional, practical, and sometimes financial support when you need it. Having a support system can help you manage stress, cope with difficult life events, and feel more connected to others.

To build a support system, start by identifying the people in your life who are most supportive and understanding. This could include family members, close friends, coworkers, or online communities. Reach out to these individuals and let them know that you value their support and would like to strengthen your relationship.

It is also helpful to seek support from mental health professionals, such as therapists or counselors, who can provide a safe and confidential space to probe your feelings and develop coping strategies. Support groups can also be valuable, as they allow you to connect with others facing similar challenges and share experiences and advice.

When building a support system, it is important to clearly communicate your needs and boundaries and be open to receiving support in different forms. This could involve asking for help with specific tasks, such as childcare or household chores, or simply venting your frustrations to a trusted friend or family member.

Remember that building a support system is an ongoing process, and finding the right people and resources to meet your needs may take time. Be patient and persistent in seeking support, and remember that you deserve to have a strong network of people who care about your well-being. Building a support system tailored to your unique needs and preferences can enhance your overall sense of connection, resilience, and self-care.

The Importance of Social Support for Women's Mental Health

Social support is essential for women's mental health and well-being. A strong network of social connections can help women cope with stress, manage emotional difficulties, and feel a sense of belonging and connectedness. A study has consistently shown that social support is linked to lower rates of depression, anxiety, and other mental health problems, as well as improved quality of life and overall health outcomes.

For women, social support can be crucial in promoting mental health. Women often face unique stressors related to gender roles, such as balancing work and family responsibilities or experiencing discrimination or violence based on gender. Social support can provide a buffer against these stressors and help women feel more empowered and resilient.

Social support can come in many forms, such as emotional support (e.g., listening and providing comfort), practical support (e.g., helping with tasks or providing resources), and informational support (e.g., sharing advice or guidance). Support can also come from various sources, including family, friends, coworkers, neighbors, and community organizations.

To build and maintain social support, it is important to prioritize relationships and engage in activities that foster connection and interaction with others. This could involve joining social clubs or groups, volunteering in the community, or regularly contacting friends or family members. It is also crucial to be open to receiving support from others and to communicate your needs and boundaries.

Overall, social support is vital to women's mental health and self-care. Women can enhance their resilience, coping skills, and overall well-being by nurturing positive relationships and cultivating a strong support network.

How to Build and Maintain Supportive Relationships

Building and maintaining supportive relationships is essential for women's mental health and well-being. Here are some tips for how to do it:

1. Be intentional: Building supportive relationships takes effort and intentionality. Make time in your schedule for socializing and nurturing relationships.

2. Be present: When spending time with others, be fully present and engaged. Put away your phone, and focus on the person you're with.

3. Be authentic: Genuineness is key to building strong relationships. Be yourself, and be willing to share your thoughts, feelings, and experiences with others.

4. Listen actively: Good communication is essential for building supportive relationships. Practice active listening by giving your full attention to the person you're talking to and seeking to understand their perspective.

5. Offer support: Be willing to offer emotional, practical, or other help when needed. This could involve offering to help with a task, providing a listening ear, or simply checking in on a friend going through a difficult time.

6. Practice empathy: Empathy is the ability to comprehend and share the feelings of others. Practice empathy by putting yourself in others' shoes and trying to see things from their perspective.

7. Set boundaries: It's essential to set boundaries in relationships to meet your needs and well-being. Be clear about what you're comfortable with, and communicate your boundaries with others.

8. Practice forgiveness: No one is perfect, and conflicts and misunderstandings are bound to happen in any relationship. Practice forgiveness by letting go of grudges and seeking to repair relationships when conflicts arise.

Building and maintaining supportive relationships takes time and effort, but it is well worth it for your mental health and well-being. By prioritizing relationships and practicing good communication and empathy, you can create a strong support network to help you navigate life's challenges and enhance your overall quality of life.

Navigating Challenging Relationships and Setting Boundaries

While building and maintaining supportive relationships is important for women's mental health, it's also important to recognize when a relationship may be more challenging or even toxic. Navigating challenging relationships can be difficult, but setting and maintaining boundaries can help.

Boundaries are limits you set for yourself in relationships to protect your well-being and ensure your needs are met. They can involve limiting your time with someone, what behaviors you will and will not tolerate, and what types of conversations you are comfortable having. Here are some tips for setting and maintaining boundaries:

1. Be clear: It's important to be clear and direct when setting boundaries. Use "I" statements to express your needs and limits, and be specific about unacceptable behaviors.

2. Stick to your boundaries: Once you've set boundaries, it's important to stick to them. This may involve saying no to requests beyond your limits or enforcing consequences if your boundaries are crossed.

3. Communicate openly: Good communication is essential for maintaining healthy boundaries. Keep the communication sequences open with the person you're

setting boundaries with, and be willing to listen to their perspective.

4. Practice self-care: Setting and maintaining boundaries can be challenging, so prioritizing self-care is important. Make time for actions that bring you joy, help you relax, and seek support from others when needed.

5. Seek professional help: If you're struggling to set or maintain boundaries in a relationship or feel like the relationship is negatively impacting your mental health, it may be helpful to seek professional help from a therapist or counselor.

It's important to recognize that setting boundaries may not always be easy and may involve difficult conversations or even ending a relationship.

However, prioritizing your own well-being and mental health is essential. By setting and maintaining healthy boundaries, you can build supportive, respectful, and beneficial relationships for your mental health.

Chapter 5: Seeking Professional Help

Seeking professional help for mental health concerns is important in taking care of your well-being. While self-care practices such as exercise, meditation, and journaling can be helpful, they may not be sufficient for everyone. If you are struggling with mental health challenges impacting your daily life, seeking professional help can provide additional support and resources.

Many mental health professionals, including therapists, psychologists, psychiatrists, and counselors, can provide support. Each of these professionals has unique training and expertise, so it's important to research and find the right fit for you.

When seeking professional help, being honest and open about your mental health concerns is important. This may involve sharing personal information and emotions that can be difficult to discuss. However, honesty and openness can help your mental health professional understand your needs and provide the most effective treatment.

Professional help may involve individual or group therapy, medication, or a combination of both. Therapy can help you develop coping strategies and build skills to manage mental health challenges. Medication can help alleviate symptoms of depression, anxiety, and other mental health concerns.

Remember that seeking professional help for mental health concerns is not a sign of weakness. It takes bravery and strength to reach out for support, which is crucial in taking care of your mental health. If you are unsure where to start, talk to your primary care physician or a trusted friend or family member who can provide guidance and support.

When to Seek Professional Help

Knowing when to seek professional help for mental health concerns can be challenging. While everyone experiences ups and downs in their mental health, it can be difficult to determine when symptoms are severe enough to warrant professional intervention.

One general rule of thumb is to seek professional help if your mental health symptoms impact your daily life and activities. If your symptoms interfere with your work, relationships, or ability to care for yourself, it may be time to seek professional help.

Some common signs that you may need professional help include the following:

1. Feeling sad or anxious for an extended period.
2. Experiencing frequent mood swings or extreme emotions.
3. Having trouble sleeping or sleeping too much.
4. Losing interest in activities you used to enjoy.
5. Feeling overwhelmed or unable to cope with stressors.
6. Having trouble concentrating or making decisions.
7. Experiencing changes in appetite or weight.
8. Having thoughts of self-harm or suicide.

It's important to remember that seeking professional help is not a sign of weakness and that many people benefit from professional support at some point. In fact, seeking help early on can lead to better outcomes and a faster recovery.

If you are unsure whether or not to seek professional help, contact a trusted friend or family member for support and guidance. You can also talk to your primary care physician or a mental health professional for an assessment and recommendations.

Different Types of Mental Health

Many mental health conditions can impact a person's well-being and quality of life. Some of the most common types of mental health conditions include:

1. Anxiety disorders are characterized by disproportionate worry, fear, or apprehension. Anxiety disorders can take many forms, including generalized anxiety disorder, panic disorder, and phobias.

2. Mood disorders: Mood disorders affect a person's emotional state, such as depression, bipolar disorder, and seasonal affective disorder.

3. Personality disorders: Personality disorders affect a person's way of thinking, feeling, and relating to others. Examples of personality disturbances include borderline personality disorder, narcissistic personality disorder, and antisocial personality disorder.

4. Eating disorders: Eating disorders involve abnormal eating habits and behaviors, such as anorexia nervosa, bulimia nervosa, and binge eating disorder.

5. Substance use disorders: Substance use disorders involve the misuse of drugs or alcohol and can range from mild to severe. Addiction is an example of a severe substance use disorder.

6. Psychotic disorders: Psychotic disorders involve changes in a person's perception of reality, such as hallucinations or delusions. Schizophrenia is an example of a psychotic disorder.

7. Trauma-related disorders are conditions triggered by a traumatic event, such as post-traumatic stress disorder (PTSD).

It's important to remember that mental health conditions are complex and can vary widely in severity and presentation. If you are encountering symptoms of a mental health condition, it's important to seek professional help for an accurate diagnosis and appropriate treatment. With the right care and support, many people can manage their mental health conditions and improve their quality of life.

Professionals and Treatments

Many different types of professionals and treatments are available to help individuals with mental health conditions. Here are some of the most common:

1. Mental health professionals: These professionals specialize in diagnosing and treating mental health conditions. Examples include psychiatrists, psychologists, social workers, and licensed therapists.

2. Medication: Many mental health conditions can be treated with medication. Psychiatric medications, such as antidepressants, antipsychotics, and mood stabilizers, can help regulate brain chemistry and reduce symptoms.

3. Therapy: Many different types of therapy can effectively treat mental health conditions. Examples include cognitive-behavioural therapy, dialectical behaviour therapy, and psychodynamic therapy.

4. Support groups: Support groups provide a space for individuals with similar experiences to come together and support each other. They can be especially helpful for those with conditions like addiction or PTSD.

5. Hospitalization: Sometimes, hospitalization may be necessary for individuals experiencing a mental health crisis. This can provide a safe and supportive environment for stabilization and treatment.

It's important to work with a mental health professional to determine the best course of treatment for your individual needs. Treatment may involve a combination of medication, therapy, and other supportive interventions. With the right care and support, it's possible to manage mental health conditions and improve the overall quality of life.

Finding the Right Provider and Getting the Most out of Therapy

Finding the right mental health provider and getting the most out of therapy can be crucial for successfully treating mental health conditions. Here are some tips:

1. Research providers: Look for mental health professionals who specialize in the specific condition or issue you're experiencing. Read online reviews, ask for referrals from friends or your primary care physician, and check your insurance provider's list of covered providers.

2. Consider the therapeutic relationship: The relationship between you and your therapist can play a big role in treatment success. It's important to find someone who you feel comfortable with and who you can trust. Consider scheduling an initial consultation to understand their approach and style.

3. Ask questions: Don't be afraid to ask about a provider's qualifications, experience, and treatment approach. It's important to feel confident in their ability to provide effective treatment.

4. Be honest: To get the most out of therapy, it's important to be honest and open with your therapist. This can be

difficult, especially when discussing sensitive or painful topics, but it's essential for making progress.

5. Set goals: Work with your therapist to set specific, achievable goals for treatment. This can help keep you focused and motivated and provide a sense of accomplishment as you progress.

6. Stay engaged: It's important to actively participate in therapy and be willing to try new strategies and techniques. This may involve completing homework assignments or practising new skills outside therapy sessions.

Finding the right provider and treatment approach may take trial and error. Don't be discouraged if the first provider or treatment approach you try doesn't work out – keep trying until you find what works for you.

Chapter 6: Overcoming Common Mental Health Challenges

Overcoming common mental health challenges can be a difficult and ongoing process, but it is possible with the right resources, support, and tools. Here are some tips on how to overwhelm common mental health challenges:

1. Develop coping skills: Coping skills are techniques and strategies that can help you manage and reduce symptoms of mental health challenges. Some examples include deep breathing exercises, mindfulness meditation, journaling, or a creative hobby.

2. Seek support: Support from loved ones, peers, or mental health professionals can be crucial in overcoming mental health challenges. Consider joining a support group or therapy group, talking to a trusted friend or family member, or seeking the help of a mental health professional.

3. Practice self-care: Self-care activities, such as exercise, healthy eating, getting enough sleep, and engaging in relaxation techniques, can help you feel more balanced and centred, which can, in turn, help you manage mental health challenges.

4. Consider medication: Medication can be an effective treatment option for some mental health challenges,

such as depression or anxiety. Talk to your healthcare provider about whether medication might be a helpful addition to your treatment plan.

5. Address underlying issues: Sometimes, mental health challenges can be symptoms of underlying issues, such as trauma, grief, or relationship problems. Addressing these underlying issues through therapy or other interventions can help improve mental health symptoms.

6. Stay engaged in treatment: Consistent engagement in treatment, whether through therapy, medication management, or support groups, can be an important factor in overcoming mental health challenges. Remember, trying different approaches is okay until you find what works best for you.

Overcoming mental health challenges can be a long and difficult journey, but with patience, persistence, and the right support, leading a fulfilling and meaningful life is possible.

Anxiety and Depression

Anxiety and depression are two considerably familiar mental health disorders affecting people today. Anxiety is a feeling of unease, worry, or fear that can be mild or severe and may be triggered by specific situations or be a constant presence in everyday life. Depression, on the other hand, is a mood disorder that can cause feelings of sadness, hopelessness, and a loss of interest in activities that were once enjoyable.

Both anxiety and depression can interfere with daily life and make it difficult to complete even simple tasks. They can affect sleep, appetite, and energy levels, leading to physical symptoms such as headaches and stomach issues.

While everyone experiences anxiety and sadness occasionally, it's important to recognize when these feelings become chronic or significantly impact daily life. If left untreated, anxiety and depression can worsen over time and may even lead to suicidal thoughts or behaviours.

Treatment options for anxiety and depression may include therapy, medication, or a combination of both. In therapy, a trained mental health professional can help individuals identify and work through the underlying causes of their anxiety or depression and develop coping skills to manage symptoms. Medications such as antidepressants or anti-anxiety drugs can also effectively reduce symptoms.

It's important to remember that seeking help for anxiety and depression is a sign of strength, not weakness. With the right approval and treatment, individuals can learn to manage their symptoms and live fulfilling, healthy lives.

Trauma and PTSD

Trauma is a distressing or disturbing event that overwhelms an individual's coping ability. Traumatic experiences can take many forms, including physical, emotional, or sexual abuse, accidents, natural disasters, or exposure to violence or war. The effects of trauma can be long-lasting and can impact a person's mental health, relationships, and overall quality of life.

Post-traumatic stress disorder (PTSD) is a mental health disorder that can develop after individual experiences or witnesses a traumatic event. Symptoms of PTSD can include re-experiencing the traumatic event through flashbacks or nightmares, avoiding reminders of the event, feeling emotionally numb or detached from others, and experiencing heightened anxiety or a sense of being constantly on edge.

PTSD can be debilitating, interfering with daily life and making it difficult to function normally. Treatment options for PTSD may include therapy, medication, or a combination of both. In therapy, a mental health professional can help individuals process the traumatic event, develop coping skills to manage symptoms, and work towards healing and recovery. Pharmaceuticals such as antidepressants or anti-anxiety drugs may also effectively reduce symptoms.

It's important to recognize that seeking help for trauma and PTSD is a brave and important step towards healing. With the right aid and remedy, individuals can learn to manage their symptoms, find a sense of safety and security, and move forward.

Substance Abuse and Addiction

Substance misuse is using drugs or alcohol in a way that can lead to physical, psychological, or social harm. It can start as experimentation but can quickly develop into addiction. Addiction is a chronic, often relapsing brain disease that causes compulsive drug seeking and use despite the harmful consequences.

Substance abuse and addiction can significantly impact an individual's mental health, relationships, and overall well-being. It can lead to physical health problems, financial difficulties, legal issues, and a range of mental health issues, including depression, anxiety, and psychosis.

Treatment options for substance abuse and addiction can vary depending on the individual's needs and the severity of the addiction. In some cases, detoxification and medical supervision may be necessary to manage withdrawal symptoms. Behavioural therapies, such as cognitive-behavioural therapy and motivational interviewing, can also be effective in helping individuals understand and change their behaviours related to substance use. Authorization groups, such as Alcoholics Anonymous or Narcotics Anonymous, can provide individuals with community support.

It's important to remember that substance abuse and addiction are treatable conditions. Seeking help and support is the first step towards recovery. With the right treatment and support, individuals can learn to manage their addiction, regain control over their lives, and move forward in their recovery journey.

Eating Disorders

Eating disorders are severe mental health conditions that involve disturbances in eating behaviours, body image, and self-esteem. They can affect people of all ages, genders, and backgrounds but are most commonly diagnosed in young women.

Several types of eating disorders include anorexia nervosa, bulimia nervosa, and binge eating disorder. Anorexia nervosa is characterized by extreme weight loss, a distorted body image, and an intense fear of gaining weight. Bulimia nervosa applies a cycle of binge eating followed by purging behaviours, such as vomiting or using laxatives. Binge eating disorder involves eating large quantities of food in a short period, often in secret and without control.

Eating disorders can have serious physical and emotional consequences, including malnutrition, dehydration, electrolyte imbalances, heart problems, and anxiety and depression. They can also be life-threatening if left untreated.

Treatment for eating disorders often involves a combination of medical management, psychotherapy, and nutrition counselling. Medications may be prescribed to address co-occurring mental health conditions, such as anxiety or depression. Psychotherapy can help individuals identify and change negative thoughts and behaviours related to food and body image. Nutrition counselling can provide education and support for developing healthy eating habits and restoring weight and nutritional balance.

It's important to seek help for an eating disorder immediately. Early intervention can improve the chances of recovery and prevent long-term physical and emotional consequences. With the right treatment and support, individuals can learn to manage their eating disorders and develop healthier relationships with food and their bodies.

Other Common Mental Health Challenges Faced by Women

In addition to anxiety, depression, trauma, PTSD, substance abuse, and eating disorders, women face various other mental health challenges. These may include:

1. Bipolar Disorder: A mental health condition characterized by extreme mood swings, including manic episodes (periods of high energy, euphoria, and creativity) and depressive episodes (periods of low mood, sadness, and hopelessness). Women are more likely to encounter rapid cycling, which involves four or more mood episodes yearly.

2. Obsessive-Compulsive Disorder (OCD): A mental health condition characterized by unwanted, intrusive thoughts (obsessions) and repetitive behaviours or mental acts (compulsions) that individuals feel driven to perform in response to their obsessions. Women are more likely to experience OCD than men.

3. Postpartum Depression: A type of dismay that occurs after giving birth, affecting up to 1 in 7 women. Symptoms may include feelings of sadness, fatigue, irritability, and hopelessness.

4. Perinatal Mood and Anxiety Disorders (PMADs): A group of mental health conditions that may occur during pregnancy or the postpartum period, including

depression, anxiety, OCD, and PTSD. PMADs impact up to 1 in 5 women.

5. Chronic Illness and Chronic Pain: Women are more likely to experience chronic illnesses such as fibromyalgia, chronic fatigue syndrome, and autoimmune diseases, contributing to depression, anxiety, and other mental health challenges.

6. Sexual Dysfunction: Women may experience various sexual difficulties, including low libido, pain during intercourse, and difficulty achieving orgasm. These challenges can contribute to shame, guilt, and low self-esteem.

It's important to note that these challenges are not mutually exclusive, and individuals may experience a range of mental health concerns simultaneously. Seeking professional help can be critical in managing these challenges and improving overall mental health and well-being.

Conclusion

As we end this comprehensive guide to women's mental health and self-care, it's important to reflect on the importance of taking care of our minds and bodies. Mental health challenges are common but can be overcome with the right tools and support. Practising self-care strategies and building a support system can improve our mental health and overall well-being.

Throughout this book, we've discussed the mind-body connection, the benefits of mind-body practices, and the importance of sleep, nutrition, exercise, and hydration. We've explored self-care practices like journaling, mindfulness, and gratitude and discussed how to create a self-care plan that works for you.

We've also talked about the importance of social support, building and maintaining supportive relationships, when to seek professional help, and how to find the right provider and get the most out of therapy.

Finally, we've discussed common mental health challenges women face, including anxiety and depression, trauma and PTSD, substance abuse and addiction, and eating disorders. Understanding these challenges and seeking appropriate treatment, we can overcome them and lead healthy, fulfilling lives.

Recollect, taking care of your mental health is not a luxury. It's a necessity. By prioritizing your mental and physical well-being, you can improve your quality of life and become the best version of yourself. So, make a commitment to yourself to practice self-care and seek help when you need it. Your mind and body will thank you.

Recap of Key Takeaways

Throughout this book, we have explored the importance of mental health and self-care for women. We have discussed various mental health challenges that women may face and the barriers and stigma that can prevent them from seeking treatment.

We have also examined the mind-body connection and the benefits of mind-body practices for mental health and self-care. Additionally, we have explored various self-care strategies, including sleep, nutrition, exercise, hydration, journaling, mindfulness, and gratitude. We discussed the importance of building a support system and seeking professional help.

As we come to the end of this book, it's important to recap some of the key takeaways. First and foremost, taking care of your mental health is essential to your overall well-being. This includes recognizing and addressing mental health challenges early on and developing a self-care plan that works for you.

It's also important to remember that seeking help is a sign of strength, not weakness. Many professionals and treatments are available to help you overcome mental health challenges, and it's important to find the right provider and get the most out of therapy.

Finally, building a supportive network of family, friends, and professionals can make all the difference in mental health and self-care. Reflect that you are not alone and that there is always hope for recovery and a better future.

Thank you for abiding the time to read this book. May it serve as a guide and resource for improving mental health and self-care.

Moving Forward: Putting Your Mental Health and Self-Care First

Moving forward with your mental health and self-care requires commitment and dedication to the practices and strategies you've learned in this book. It's essential to prioritize your well-being, making it a non-negotiable aspect of your life.

To do so, it's important to reflect on the key takeaways from this book. Remember that mental health and self-care are critical for women's health and well-being. Understanding the common mental health challenges women face and seeking help when necessary is crucial.

It's also essential to recognize the mind-body connection and the benefits of mind-body practices for mental health and self-care. Building a supportive community and seeking professional help is vital to maintaining good mental health.

As you move forward, take the time to create a self-care plan that works for you, including self-care essentials like sleep, nutrition, exercise, and hydration, as well as other practices like journaling, mindfulness, and gratitude. Remember to set boundaries and navigate challenging relationships, seeking help when necessary.

Overall, putting your mental health and self-care first is a journey that requires patience, self-compassion, and dedication. But by prioritizing your well-being, you'll find that you have more energy, resilience, and happiness to live a fulfilling life.

Appendix: Additional Resources for Women's Mental Health and Self-Care

This appendix lists additional resources supporting women's mental health and self-care journey. These resources include websites, helplines, and apps that offer information, support, and tools for managing mental health.

Websites:

- National Institute of Mental Health (https://www.nimh.nih.gov/): This website provides information on mental health conditions, treatment options, and research on mental health.
- Mental Health America (https://www.mhanational.org/): This website offers resources on mental health screening, finding help, and different mental health topics.
- The Mighty (https://themighty.com/): This website provides articles and personal stories on mental health, chronic illness, and disability.

Helplines:

- National Suicide Prevention Lifeline (1-800-273-TALK): This helpline provides free and confidential support for distressed individuals, including those feeling suicidal.
- Crisis Text Line (text HOME to 741741): This helpline provides free and confidential support via text message for individuals in crisis.

- National Alliance on Mental Illness (NAMI) Helpline (1-800-950-NAMI): This helpline provides information and support for individuals with mental illness and their families.

Apps:

- Headspace: This app offers guided meditations and mindfulness exercises to help manage stress and improve mental health.
- Calm: This app provides guided meditations, sleep stories, and breathing exercises to help reduce anxiety and improve sleep.
- Moodfit: This app offers tools for tracking mood and setting goals for self-care.

These are just a few illustrations of the many resources available to support women's mental health and self-care. By seeking help and using available resources, women can improve their mental health and overall well-being.

Acknowledgement

Writing a book on mental health and self-care for women has been a challenging and rewarding experience. I would like to thank everyone who sustained me in this journey.

Preferably and best, I thank the women who shared their personal stories with me. Your courage, resilience, and strength inspired me to write this book. Your experiences and insights will help other women struggling with their mental health.

I would also like to thank my relatives and friends, who provided me with emotional support and encouragement throughout this process. Your belief in me gave me the confidence to pursue this project and see it through to completion.

I am grateful to the mental health professionals who generously shared their expertise. Your insights and guidance helped me better understand the challenges faced by women and the importance of self-care.

Finally, I want to thank my publisher and editor, who believed in this project and gave me invaluable feedback and support. Your expertise and professionalism helped me shape this book into its final form.

Thank you to everyone who contributed to bringing this book to life. Your contributions are deeply appreciated.

Index

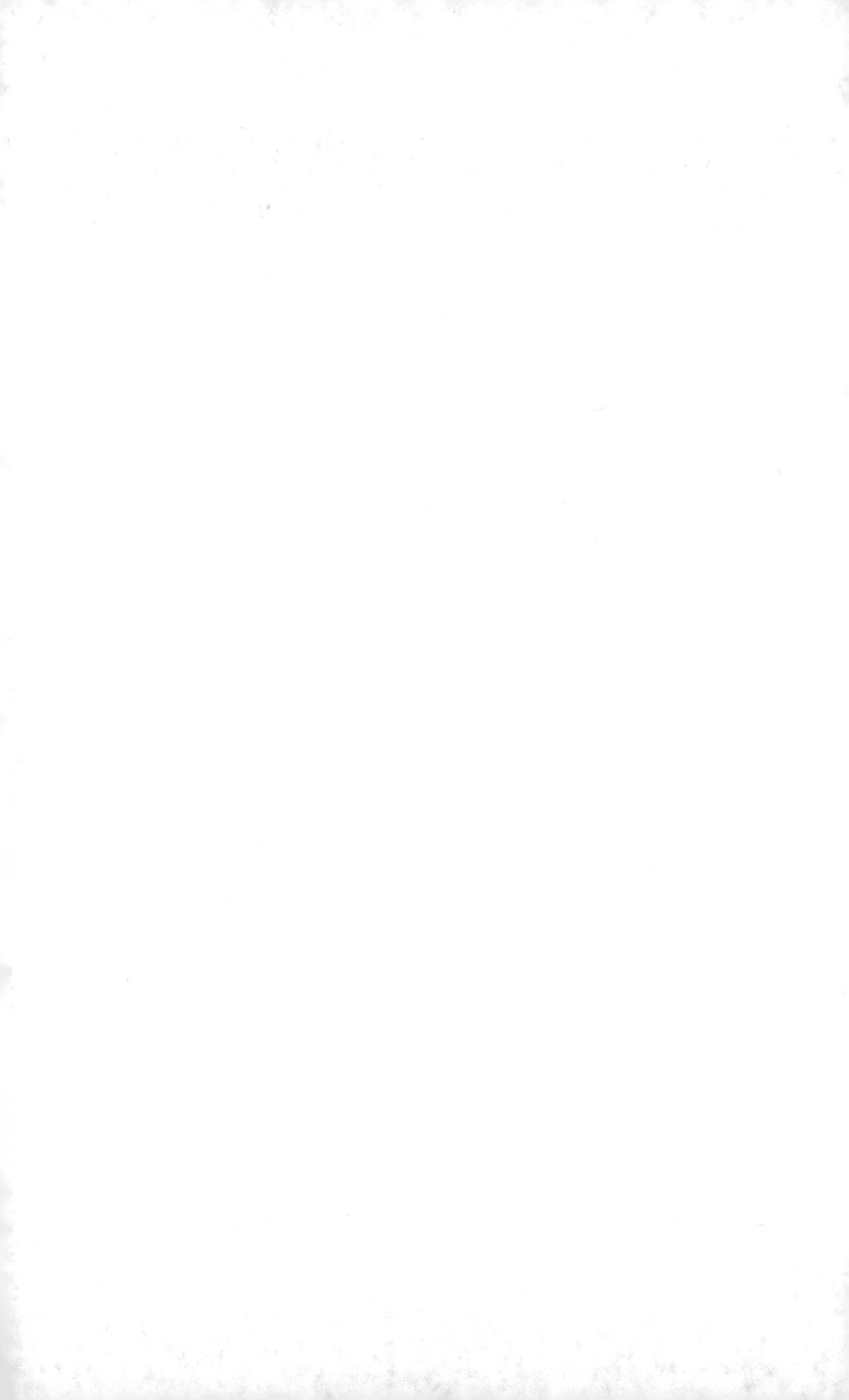